OSTEOARTHRITIS DIET HANDBOOK

A Complete Diet Plan For Osteoarthritis Patients

EMILEE MCCOY

Table of Contents

CHAPTER ONE

Diet for osteoarthritis

Osteoarthritis is a degenerative joint disease.

For many people, easing the discomfort of osteoarthritis symptoms like pain, stiffness, and swelling can be as simple as making dietary adjustments.

There are over thirty million American adults who suffer from osteoarthritis, the most common type of arthritis. It occurs as a result of the deterioration of joint cartilage over time.

Anyone can suffer from it, but it is most common in knees and hands, as well as hips and spines.

In this article, we'll examine which foods to include in the diets of people with osteoarthritis and which to avoid. We also debunk a few common myths about arthritis and food.

What role does diet play in osteoarthritis treatment?

Maintaining a healthy weight and eating a well-balanced diet can help keep joint damage at bay.

According to the Arthritis Foundation, certain diets can help alleviate osteoarthritis symptoms, but no specific foods or supplements can cure the disease.

There are foods that are anti-inflammatory and can help alleviate symptoms, while there are others that can exacerbate them.

Osteoarthritis can be improved by following a healthy diet:

Maintaining a healthy immune system and preventing injury

An osteoarthritis patient's best defense against further joint damage is a well-balanced, nutrient-dense diet.

Anti-inflammatory diets can alleviate symptoms by reducing inflammation in the body.

Antioxidants, such as vitamins A, C, and E, may help prevent further joint damage if you consume enough of them in your diet.

Cholesterol-lowering drugs

Reduced cholesterol levels may improve the symptoms of osteoarthritis in those who are at risk for the condition. Cholesterol levels can be quickly reduced with the right diet.

The goal is to keep one's weight in check.

Having too much weight on your frame can put additional strain on your joints, and having too much fat around your organs can exacerbate inflammation already present. Osteoarthritis symptoms can be reduced by maintaining a healthy weight.

In particular for those with medical conditions that limit mobility, such as osteoarthritis, it can be difficult to maintain a healthy weight. A doctor or a nutritionist will be able to give you advice on what to eat.

How and why to eat these eight foods

Bone, muscle, and joint health can be improved and inflammation and disease prevented by eating certain foods.

Osteoarthritis sufferers may find relief from their symptoms by including the eight foods listed below in their diet:

Fish high in omega-3 fatty acids

Omega-3 fatty acids, which have anti-inflammatory properties, are found in abundance in salmon.

Omega-3 fatty acids are abundant in oily fish. Osteoarthritis sufferers may benefit from the anti-inflammatory properties of these polyunsaturated fats.

It is recommended that people with osteoarthritis eat at least one serving of oily fish each week. Included in the list of "oily fish" are:

- sardines

- mackerel
- salmon
- fresh tuna

Supplements containing omega-3 fats, such as fish oil, krill oil, or flaxseed oil, are available for those who don't want to eat fish.

Chia seeds, flaxseed oil, and walnuts are all excellent sources of omega-3 fatty acids. Inflammation-fighting properties can be found in some of these foods.

CHAPTER TWO

2. Liquids

Inflammation can be reduced by other oils besides those found in oily fish. Oleocanthal, a compound found in high concentrations in extra virgin olive oil, may have anti-inflammatory properties similar to those found in nonsteroidal anti-inflammatory drugs (NSAIDs).

In addition to being good for you, avocado and safflower oils have been shown to lower cholesterol.

Dairy is the third item on the list.

There is a lot of calcium and vitamin D in dairy products like milk, yogurt and cheese. Strengthening the bones with the help of these nutrients may alleviate painful symptoms.

Milk contains proteins that can aid in muscle development. Low-fat options are available to those who want to keep their weight in check.

Intensely colored leafy greens

Vitamin D and stress-fighting phytochemicals and antioxidants are found in dark leafy greens. Vitamin D helps the body absorb calcium and boosts the immune system, allowing it to fight off disease.

The following are examples of dark leafy greens:

- spinach
- kale

- chard

- collard greens,

Broccoli is number five.

Sulforaphane, a compound found in broccoli, has been shown to slow the progression of osteoarthritis.

Vitamins K and C, as well as calcium, are also found in this vegetable.

a cup of sencha

Inflammation and damage to cartilage may be slowed by polyphenols, which are antioxidants. Polyphenols are abundant in green tea.

8. Onion

To counteract enzymes that damage cartilage, researchers believe diallyl disulfide, a component of garlic.

Nuts are number eight on the list.

Nuts are high in calcium, magnesium, zinc, vitamin E, and

fiber, all of which are beneficial to the heart. They also contain the immune system booster alpha-linolenic acid (ALA).

There's also the Mediterranean diet.

Osteoarthritis sufferers may benefit from a Mediterranean diet, which has been shown to reduce inflammation.

When it comes to weight loss, a Mediterranean-style diet can help alleviate the symptoms of osteoarthritis as well as other health issues.

A Mediterranean diet may also lower the risk of developing:

in addition to heart attacks and strokes

- Aging-related muscle wasting

- Dementia and Alzheimer's disease

Diseases such as Parkinson's

- death by natural causes

Fruits and vegetables, whole grains, legumes, fish, yogurt,

and heart-healthy fats like olive oil and nuts are all staples of the Mediterranean diet.

People's diets can be easily adapted to resemble that of the Mediterranean region by making a few simple adjustments. Some examples are as follows:

Consuming starchy foods like sweet potatoes, potatoes and beans and lentils as well as whole-grain breads and pastas

getting plenty of fresh produce into your diet

increasing the intake of fish

- Cutting back on meat consumption

- opting for products containing oils derived from plants and vegetables, like olive oil

- Choosing wholemeal over refined flour options

-

Three foods to stay away from and why

CHAPTER THREE

Inflammation can be caused by consuming processed sugars.

Osteoarthritis patients have an inflammatory state in their bodies.

Foods that have anti-inflammatory properties may help alleviate symptoms, but some foods contain substances that actually exacerbate the inflammation. The best thing to do is to avoid or limit these food choices.

Foods to steer clear of include the following:

Sugar is the first ingredient.

Sugar processing can trigger the release of cytokines, which act as the body's messengers of inflammation. For example, the added sugars found in sugared beverages such as sodas and flavored coffees are the most likely to cause inflammation.

2. Unhealthy fats

Saturated fats, such as those found in pizza and red meat, can irritate fat tissue. Additionally, this can exacerbate arthritis inflammation while increasing the risk of obesity, heart disease, and other conditions.

3. Refined carbohydrate sources

When refined carbohydrates like white bread, rice, and potato chips are consumed, AGE oxidants can be produced in large quantities. These can cause the body to become inflamed.

Dispelling three myths about arthritis-related food intolerances

Some claim that certain foods can exacerbate the symptoms of osteoarthritis, but scientific evidence is lacking.

Here are three common misconceptions:

Inflammation is caused by citrus fruits.

Some people believe that citrus fruits are inflammatory because of their acidity. Nonetheless, this is not the case. Citrus fruits are rich in vitamin C and antioxidants and have anti-inflammatory properties.

Nonetheless, some anti-arthritis medications can interact with grapefruit juice. Before incorporating it into a patient's diet, they should consult with their doctor.

Osteoarthritis can be alleviated by avoiding dairy products.

Osteoarthritis may benefit from a dairy-free diet, according to some studies. However, while some people find dairy products to be problematic, others find them to have anti-inflammatory properties.

Those with gout-related inflammatory symptoms may benefit from drinking skimmed or low-fat milk.

A dairy-free diet can help people determine whether or not their symptoms improve or worsen with the consumption of the dairy product.

Toxic effects of nightshade vegetables.

Solanine, a chemical found in solanaceous vegetables such as tomatoes, potatoes, eggplants, and peppers, has been blamed by some for causing arthritis pain. Arthritis Foundation claims that there is no evidence to support this. There are numerous health benefits to incorporating these vegetables into one's diet.

Don't forget about the power of food in your battle against knee osteoarthritis (OA). There isn't a specific diet for your condition, but smart eating can provide substantial health benefits. You'll be able to maintain a healthy weight, strengthen your cartilage, and reduce inflammation.

You don't have to drastically alter your eating habits. Maintaining healthy joints is as simple as following these simple steps.

2. Eliminate Unnecessary Fats

Keep your waistline in check and your knees will thank you. You'll put less strain on your joints if you lose weight. Reduce your calorie intake by eating smaller portions, avoiding sugary foods and beverages, and consuming a majority of your diet from plants.

Eating a Variety of Fruits and Vegetables

There's no limit to how much you can eat of these. The antioxidants found in many of these foods may be able to help protect your cells from oxidative stress.

Various fruits and vegetables, such as apples and onions, may also contain antioxidants that can reduce joint inflammation and pain.

Add Omega-3 Fatty Acids to the Diet

Joint pain and stiffness are two common side effects of a diet low in omega-3 fatty acids. These supplements work by reducing the body's inflammatory response to the stimuli they provide.

Don't forget about the power of food in your battle against knee osteoarthritis (OA). There isn't a specific diet for your condition, but smart eating can provide substantial health benefits. You'll be able to maintain a healthy weight, strengthen your cartilage, and reduce inflammation.

You don't have to drastically alter your eating habits. Maintaining healthy joints is as simple as following these simple steps.

Fatty fish can easily be added to your diet by consuming two 3-ounce servings each week. Fish such as trout, salmon, mackerel, herring, tuna, and sardines are excellent sources of omega-3 fatty acids.

As an alternative to other fats, use olive oil instead.

Oleocanthal, an olive oil compound, was found to have anti-inflammatory properties comparable to those of ibuprofen in one study. The most flavorful olive oils have the highest concentration.

Use olive oil in place of other fats, such as butter, to get the benefits of olive oil without adding calories.

The Importance of Adequate Vitamin C Intake

Collagen and connective tissue are essential components of joint health, and vitamin C is a vital component. This nutrient can be found in a wide variety of delicious foods. Make sure to eat a variety of fruits and vegetables like oranges, tangerines, berries, broccoli, cabbage and kale. Aim for the daily allowance of 75 milligrams for women and 90 milligrams for men as a general guideline.

Cooking at high temperatures should be avoided.

Compounds formed during the high-temperature cooking of meat can lead to inflammation in the body. Many diseases, including arthritis, heart disease, and type 2 diabetes, have been linked to the accumulation of these so-called advanced glycation end products (AGEs).

Reduce the amount of AGEs in your diet by avoiding foods that have been fried, grilled, broiled, or microwaved. Processed foods should also be avoided because they are frequently cooked at high temperatures.

Takeaway

Evidence suggests certain foods and nutrients help osteoarthritis sufferers. As a result, they help reduce swelling and inflammation, as well as support healthy bones, muscles, and an effective immune system.

Avoiding or restricting foods that cause inflammation may also be beneficial to some people.

As a result of being overweight or obese, the symptoms of osteoarthritis can be exacerbated.

Osteoarthritis patients who eat a diet rich in vegetables, fiber, and anti-inflammatory fats, such as the Mediterranean diet, can keep their weight in check.

Symptoms like pain and swelling will be reduced as a result.

THE END

www.ingramcontent.com/pod-product-compliance
Lightning Source LLC
Chambersburg PA
CBHW050816160726
48004CB00002B/877